Wren the Writer

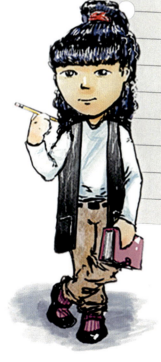

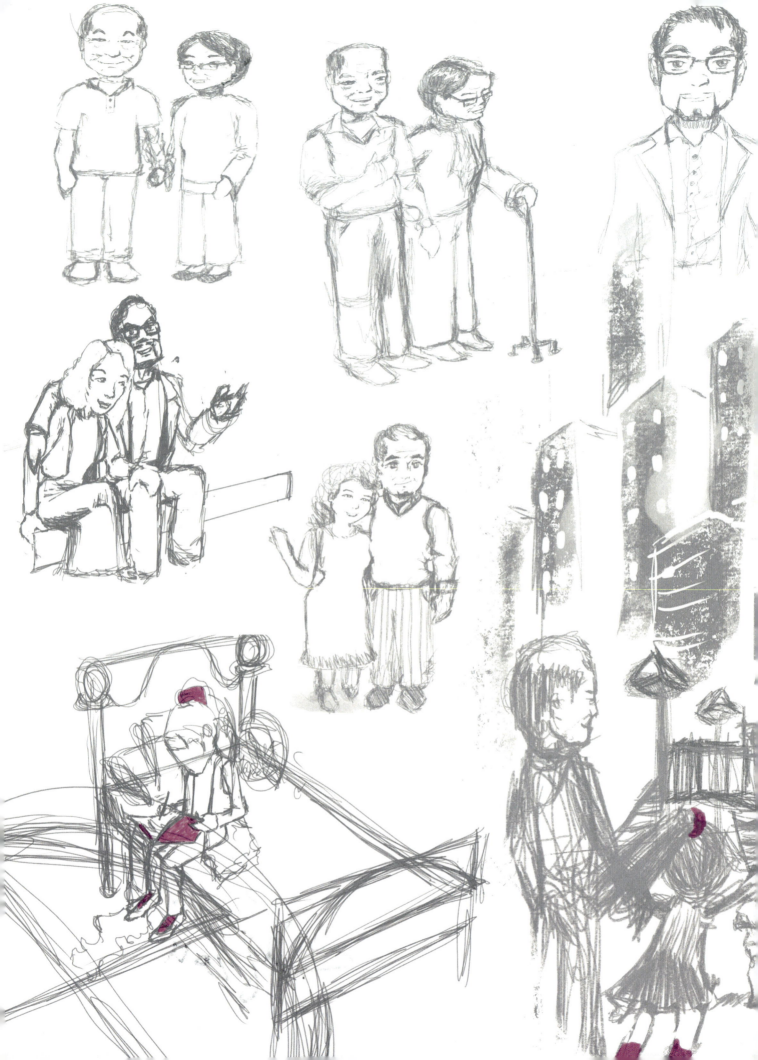

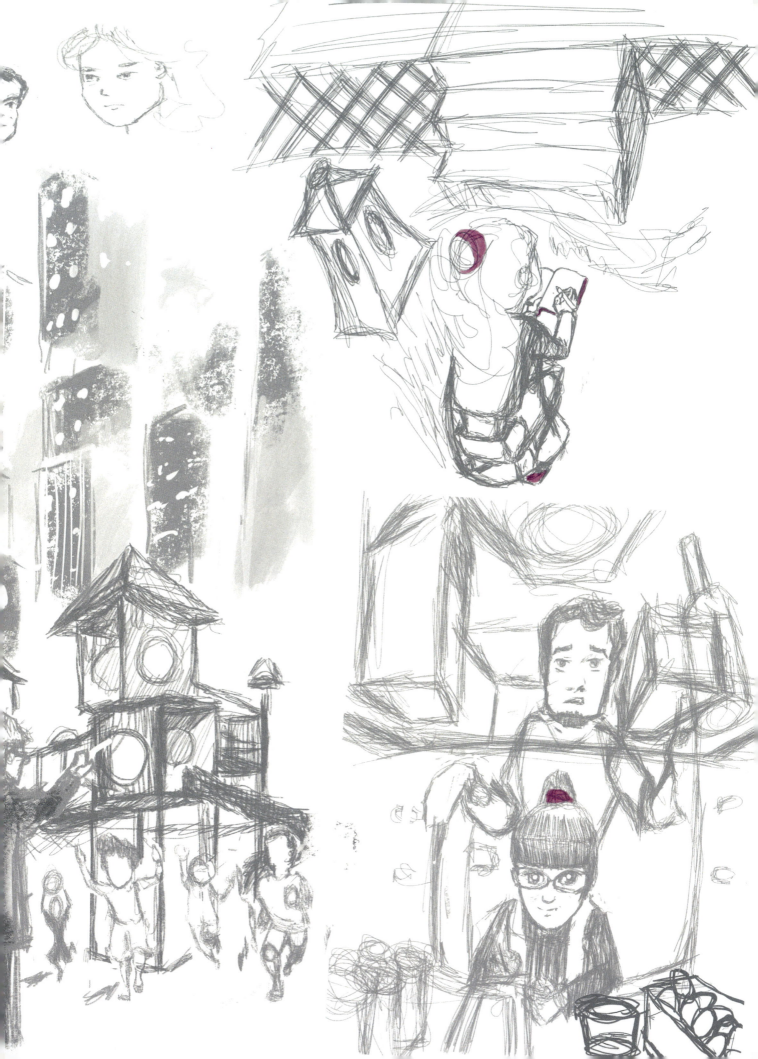

For my family and friends —
thank you for the love and support
that keeps me writing.
J. Baker-Smith

For Prince John-John and
Princess Mia — wisdom, strength,
mercy, and peace, and may the
stars dance at your feet.
J. Moorer

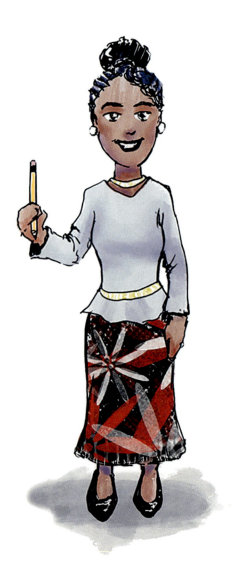

Library of Congress Cataloging-in-Publication Data is on file with the publisher.

Text copyright © 2019 by Joanne Baker-Smith
Illustrations copyright © 2019 by John Moorer
Published in 2019 by Baker-Smith Publishers and Moorerland Studios
in connection with Kindle Direct Publishing

ISBN 978-1-0955-9454-4

All rights reserved. No part of this book may be reproduced or transmitted in any form or by any means, electronic or mechanical, including photocopying, recording, or by any information storage and retrieval system, without the written permission of the publisher.

Printed in the United States

Design and composition by Sophie Appel

Wren the Writer

By Joanne Baker-Smith

Illustrated by John Moorer

LITTLE LEARNER SERIES · BOOK TWO

Wren sat on the rug with her classmates, happily waiting for her teacher to begin.

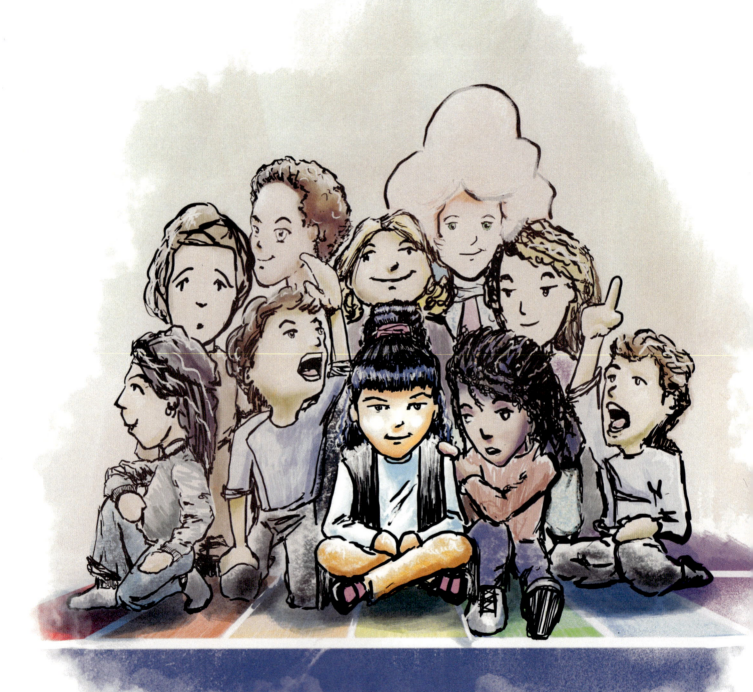

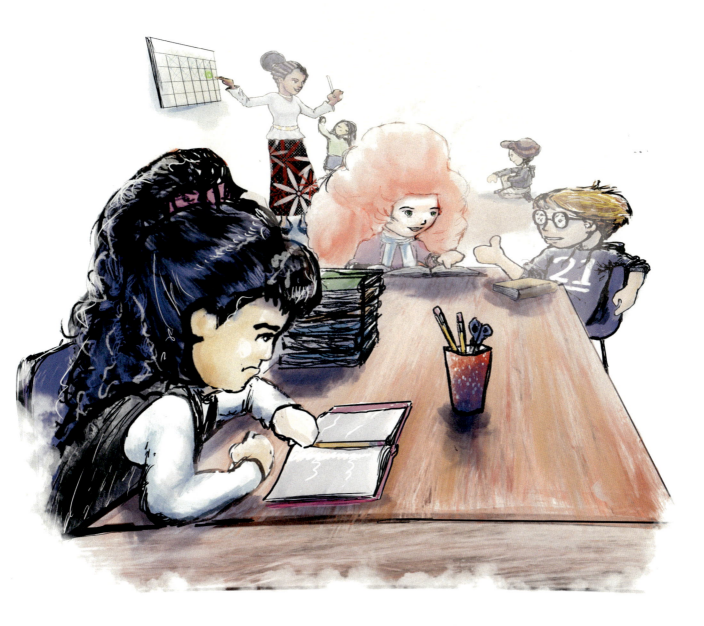

"Tomorrow we will start our first writing unit!" Ms. Smith said with a smile. Wren loved reading, but she was a little nervous about writing. She didn't exactly feel like a writer.

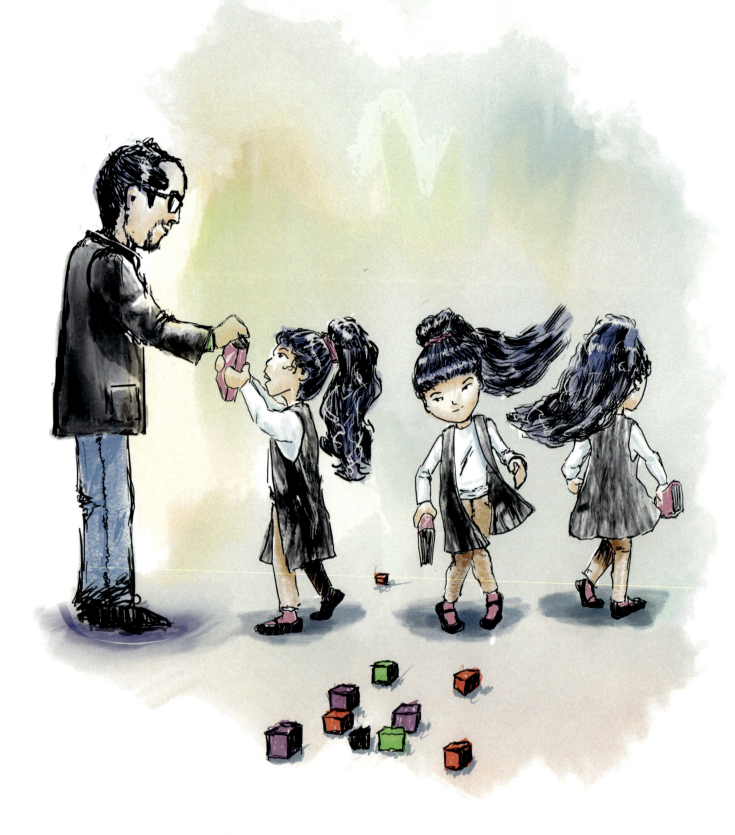

Later that day when her dad picked her up from After School, she told him how she felt about the new writing unit.

Her dad smiled and confidently said,
"You can do this, you're a writer!"
Wren looked at her father curiously.

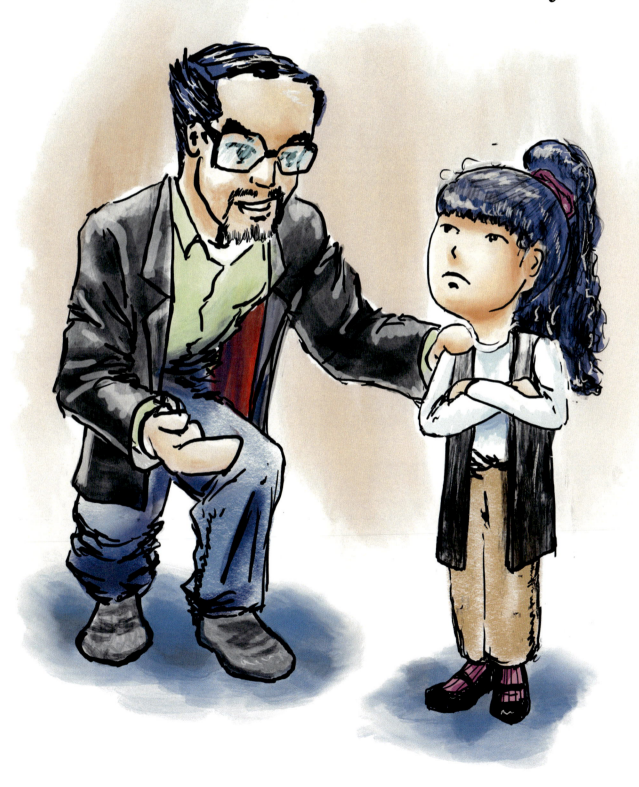

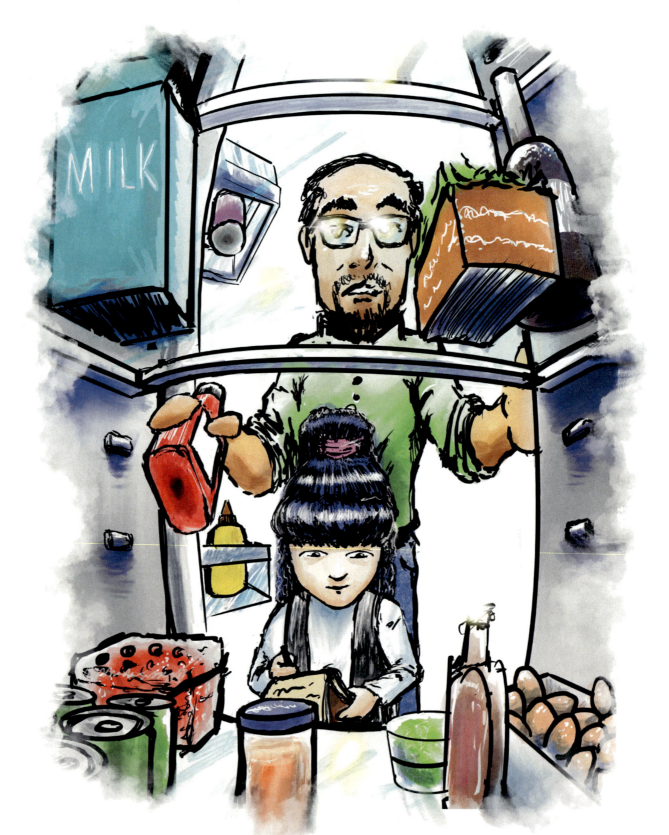

"You are always the first to help me write lists when I need to remember what to get at the grocery store," her father said.

"That's right! I also write lists of my favorite things in my unicorn notebook," Wren added.

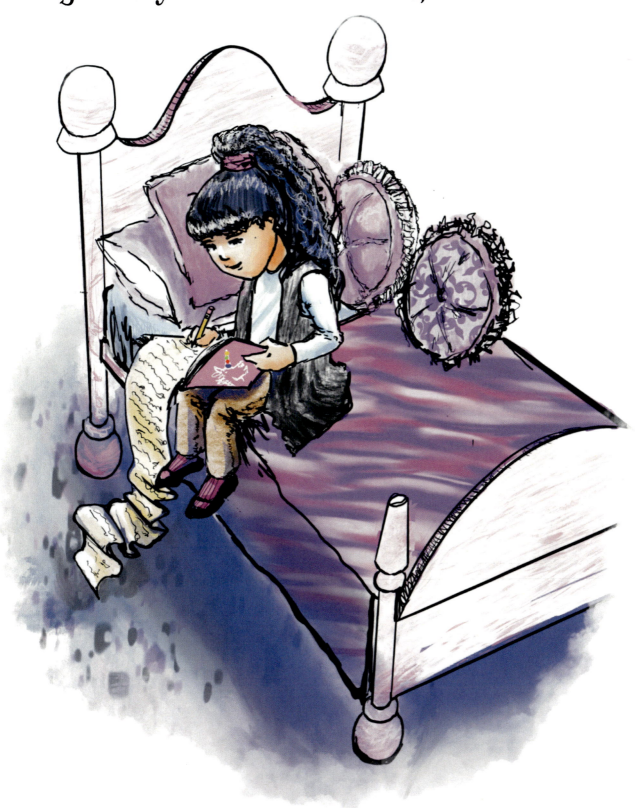

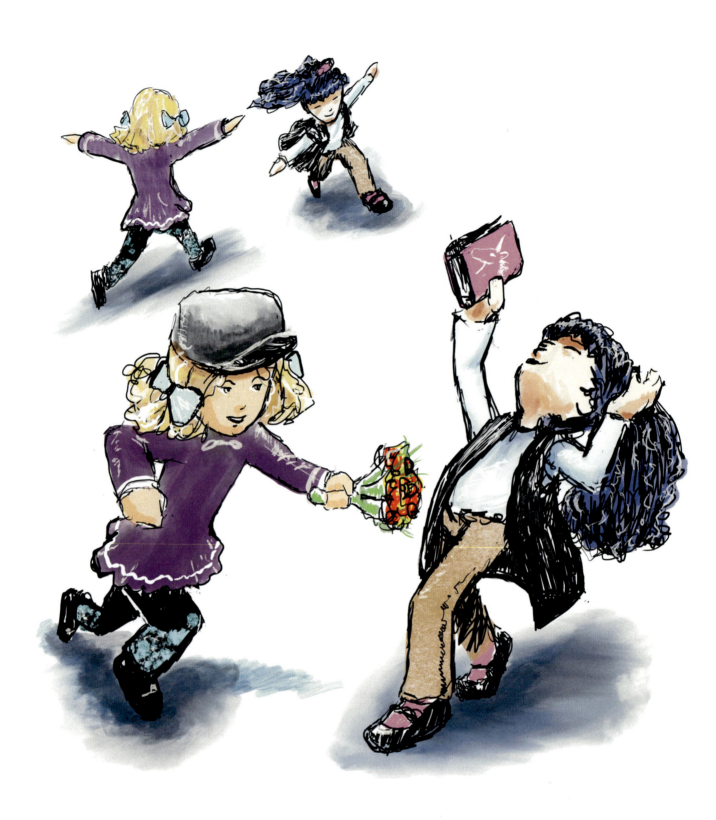

"You and Norah can spend a whole afternoon making up stories and writing plays," he noted.

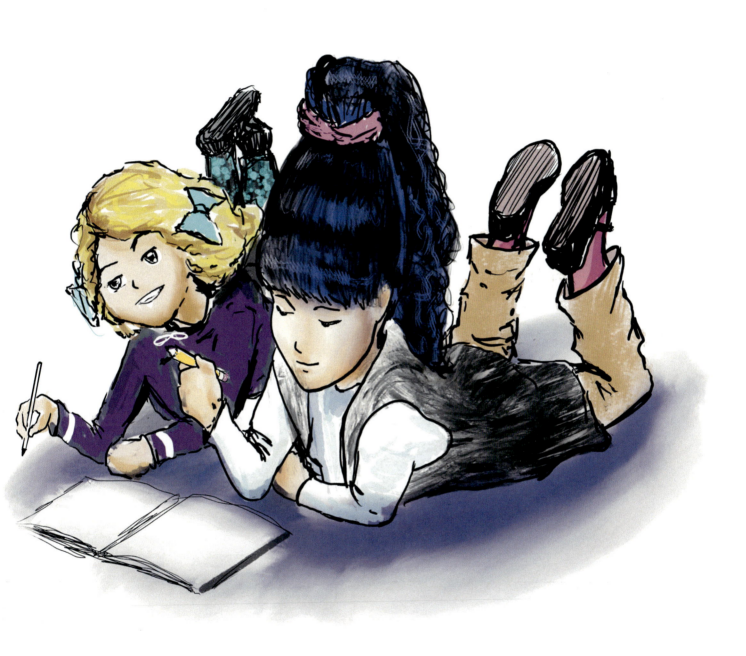

Wren grinned and added,
"Norah writes a sentence and then I add one."

"When you, Grandma, and Grandpa go to the park, you three are always writing down the interesting things you notice," her dad continued.

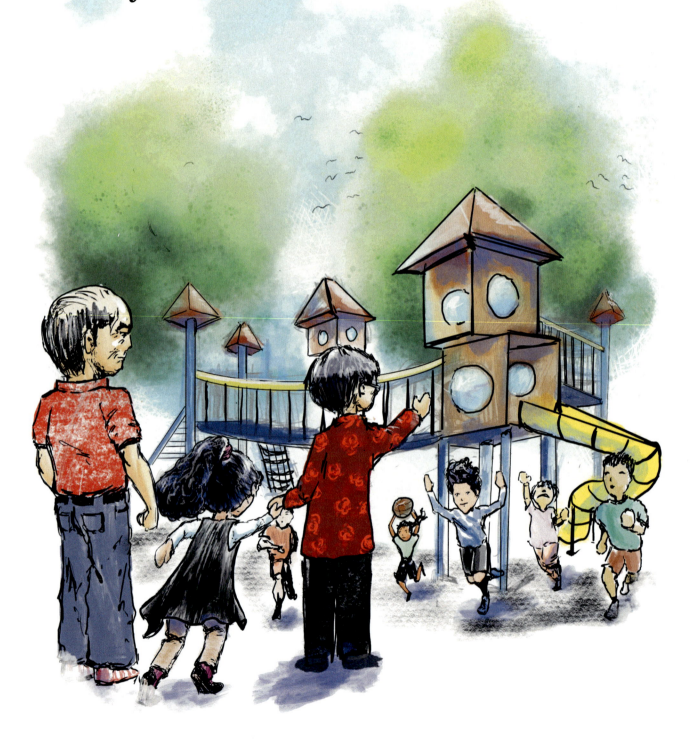

"Last week we saw a beautiful blue jay sitting in a tree," Wren said with a smile.

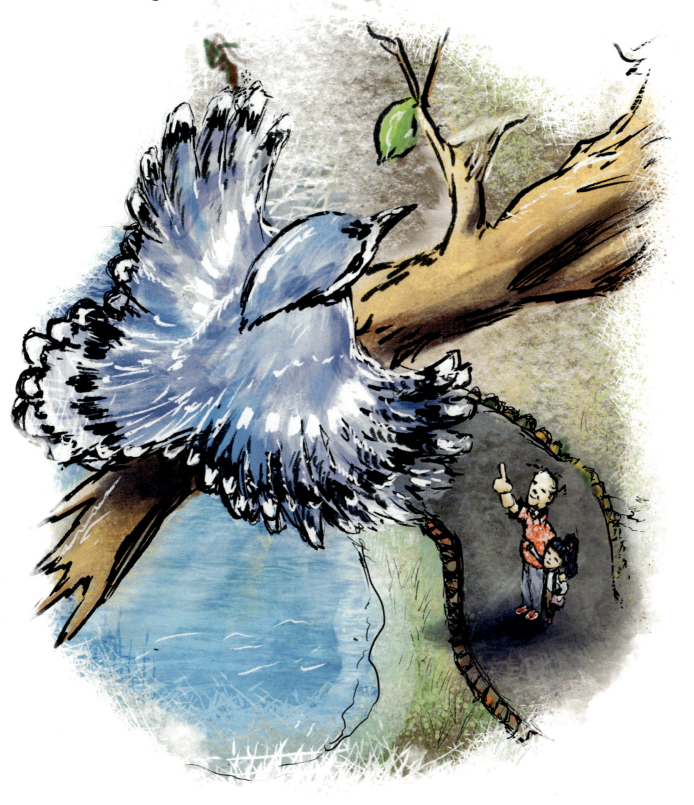

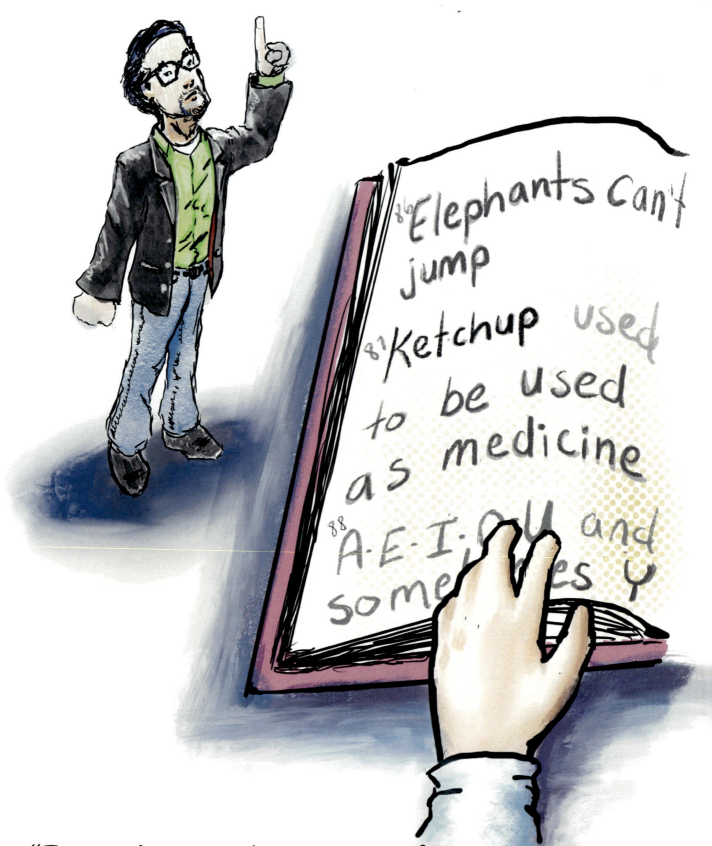

"Every time you learn a new fact you write it down and add it to our Interesting Fact List," Dad pointed out.

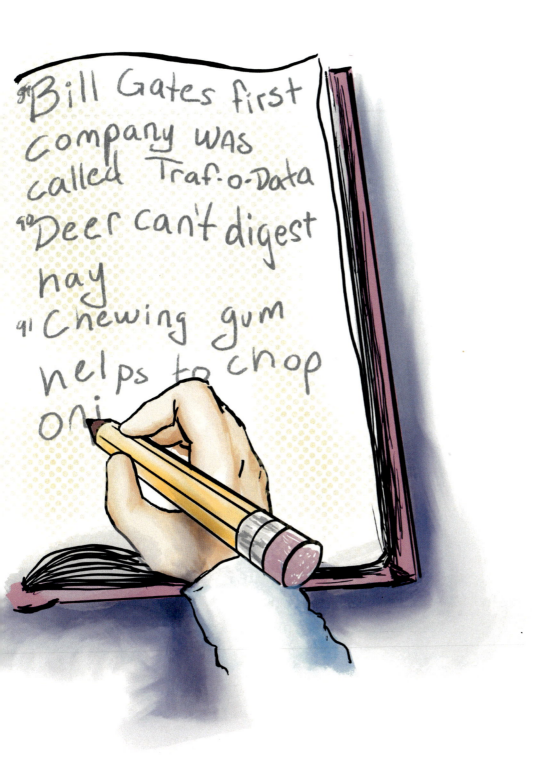

"We almost have 100 facts," Wren exclaimed.

"And what about that wonderful collection of interesting words you have in your word jar?" Dad asked.

"It's fun to collect new words, especially when they are fun to say," Wren smiled with delight.

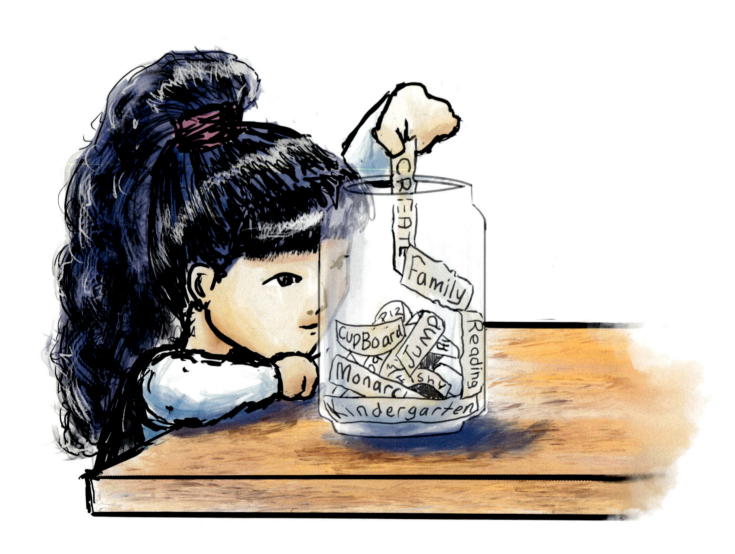

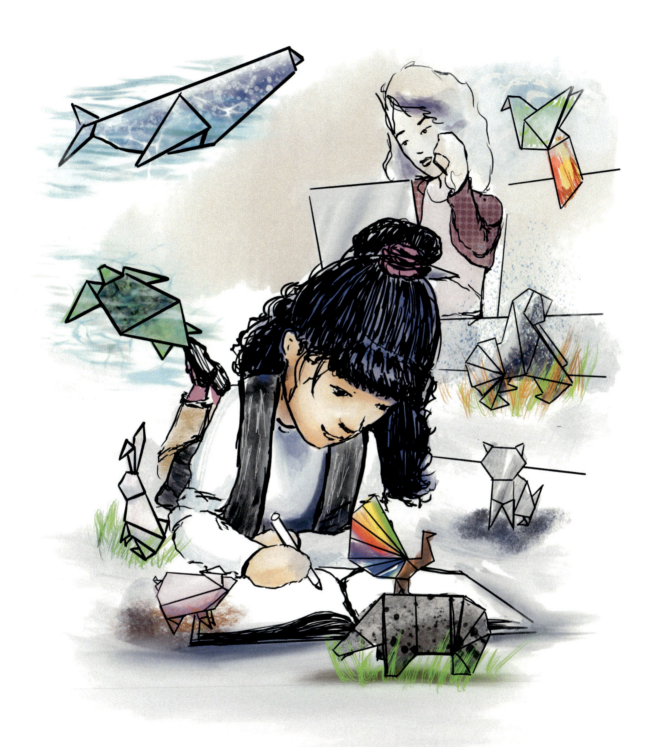

"And don't forget your beautiful drawings. I love the way you label them and write stories to go with them," Dad beamed with pride.

"You are
a writer!"
said Dad.

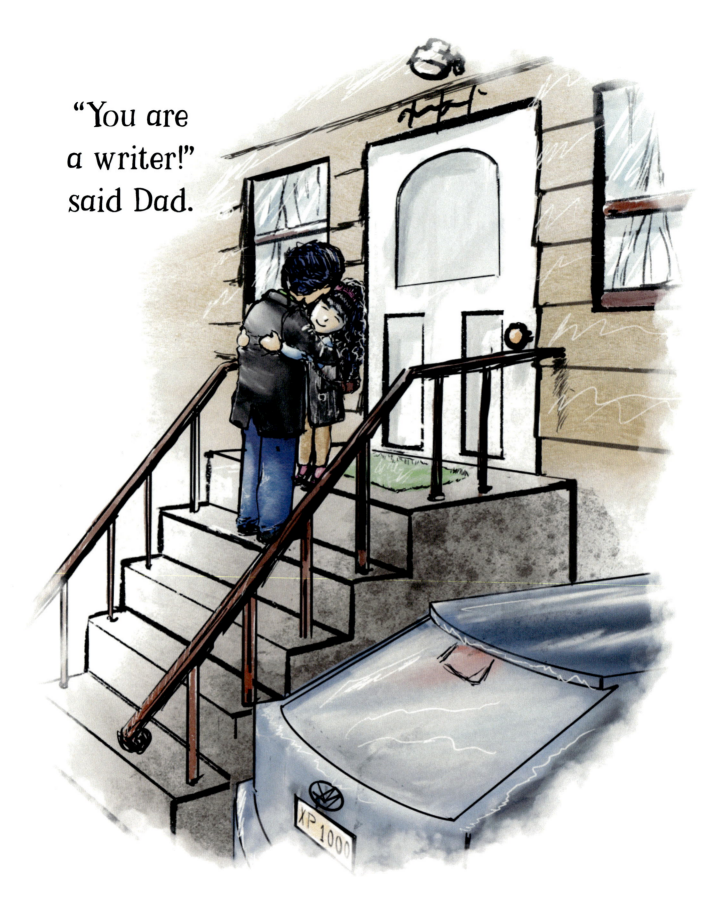

Wren hugged her dad tightly.
"Thanks, Dad!" Wren sweetly sang.

When they got home, Wren quickly said hello to her mom and brother as she dashed past them to get her unicorn notebook.

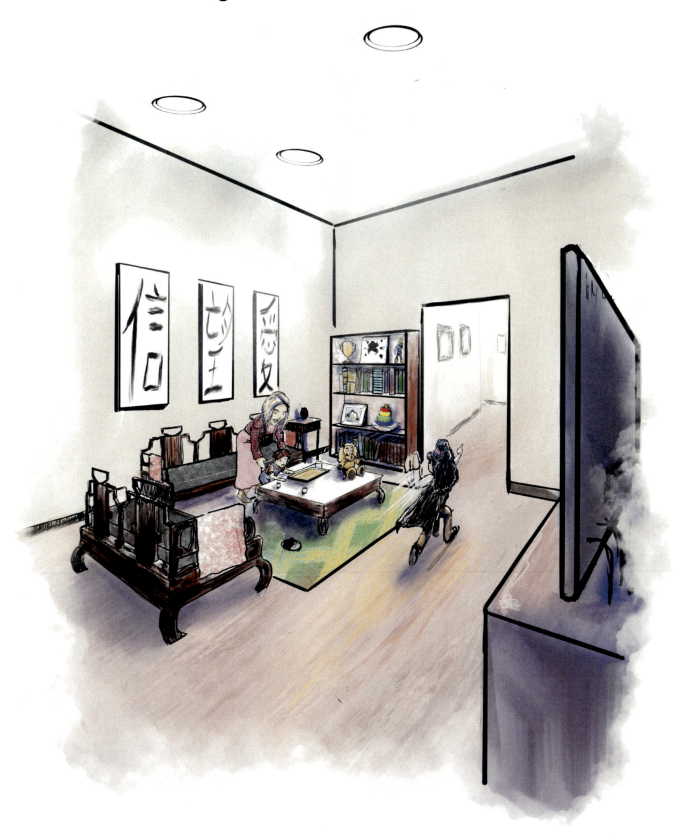

She came back and said to her parents, "I am going in the yard to see what I notice."

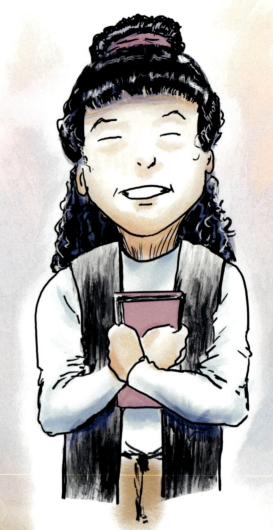

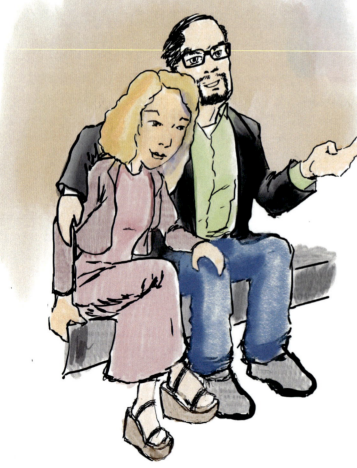

"Spoken like a true writer," her dad said with a smile.

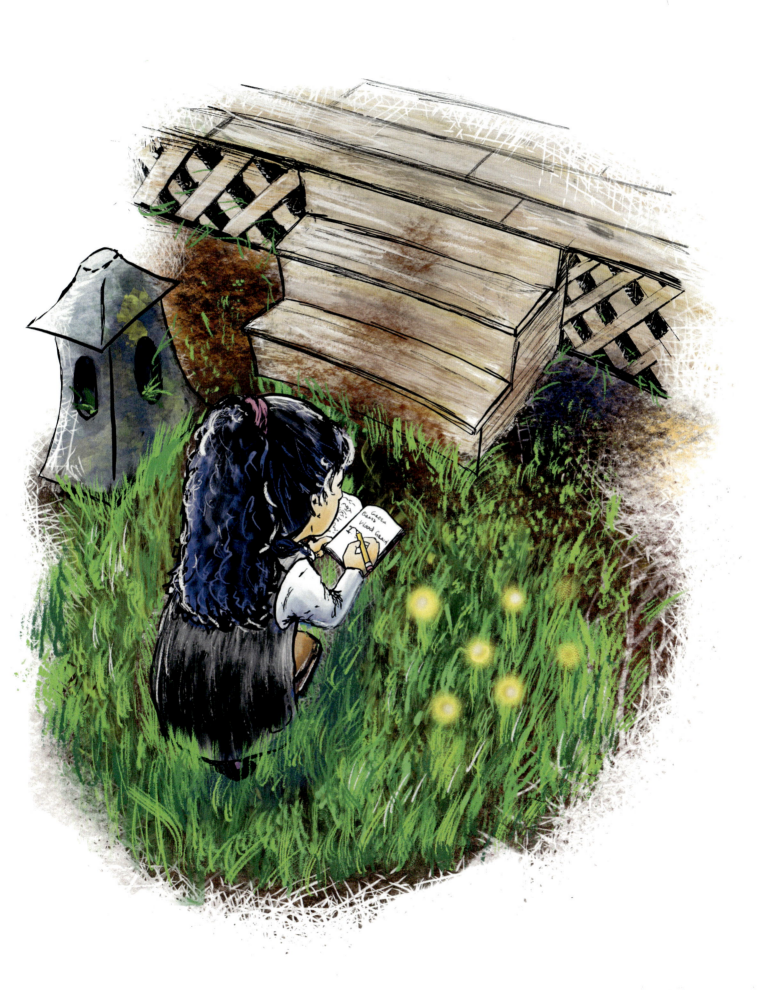

The next day during writing time, Wren smiled when her teacher began to discuss their writing unit.

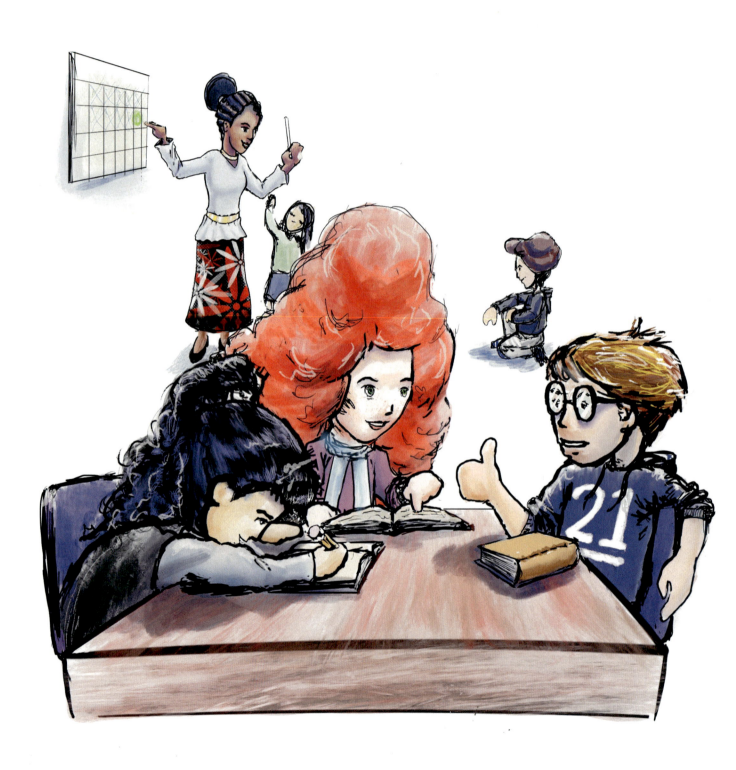

"I'm ready for this!" Wren said to herself as she walked back to her desk to get started on her idea web.

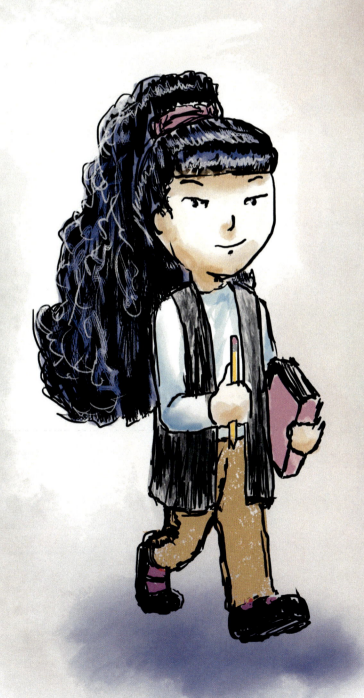

When the writing period was over, Wren looked down at her paper and quietly said, 'This is going to be a great story!"

Her teacher leaned over and whispered, "I agree!"

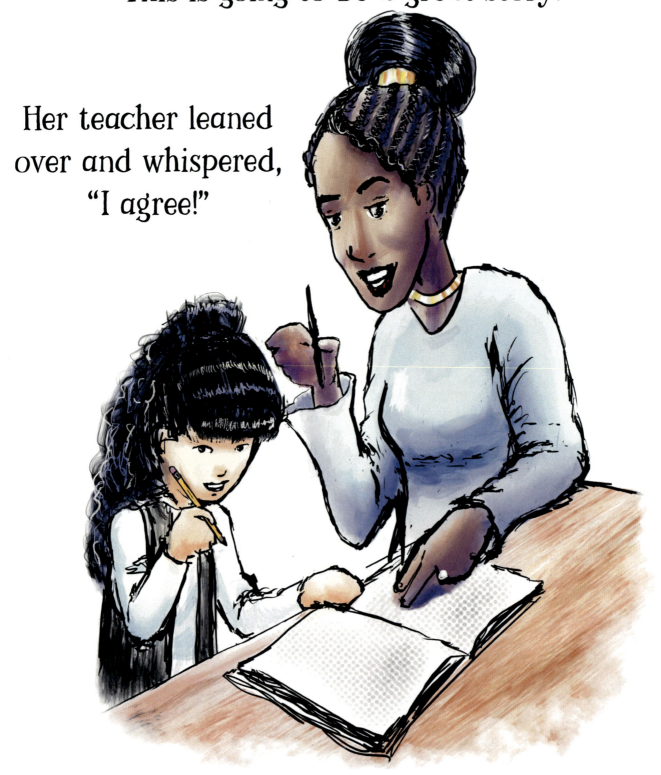

Wren couldn't wait to get home
and tell her family all about the story
she was going to write.

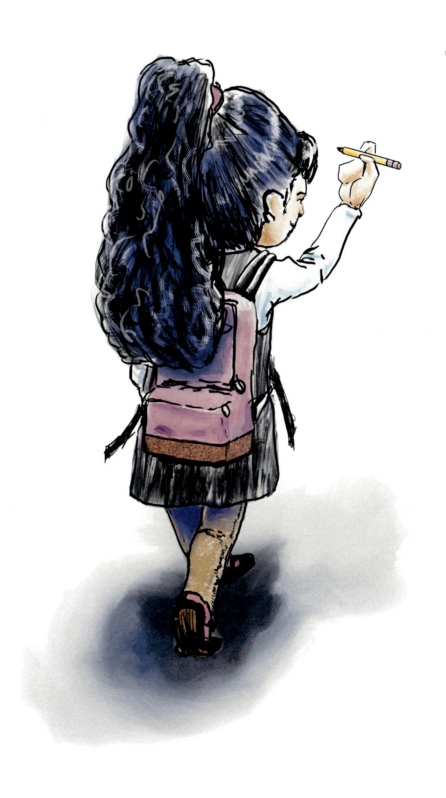

Writer's Pages

Now that you have finished Wren the Writer, get out there and write! Here are some great ways to grow as a writer.

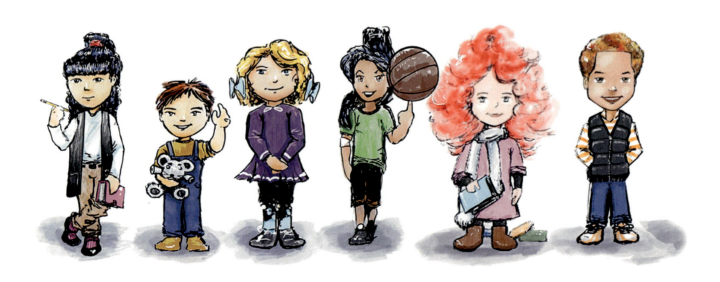

— Gathering Ideas —

Writers are constantly gathering ideas. Start a notebook and fill it with...

Lists — write lists of your favorite places, people, foods, colors, etc.

Observations — sit in your home, the park, the bus and write all that you notice (a green wiggly plant, a friendly child with a sparkly blue shirt, the birds chirping, etc.)

Interesting Facts — gather facts from books you read or have read to you, from your favorite television shows, from trips to the zoo or museums, from your family or teachers.

— Generate Details —

Writers write with detail.
Take one of your ideas from
your notebook and describe it.

Sensory Words — Use your 5 senses to describe your favorite place, things you notice in your home, or a fact you learned.

What do you see? (color, shape, size, etc.)
What do you feel? (rough, bumpy, smooth, etc.)
What do you taste? (sweet, sour, sugary, etc.)
What do you hear? (silence, buzzing, rattling, etc.)
What do you smell? (fragrant roses, stinky garbage, etc.)

Sketch it out –
draw out the memory or moment
you are trying to describe.
Be sure to write a sentence or 2
about each item you include
in your drawing.

Thoughts & Feelings –
Remember to tell what you were feeling
(excited, exhausted, confused) and why.
Include your thoughts as well. Tell what
you were thinking ("Is this for real?,"
I thought to myself.)

Word Wizards

Words are magical! Gather as many as you can!

Word Collection Jars/Walls

When you or a family member hear an interesting, funny, or new word, write it down and either put it in a jar or on a designated collection wall. Share your new-found words with each other and see if you can use them throughout your day.

Personal Dictionary

Create your own dictionary by writing new words in a notebook along with their meaning. You can organize them anyway you want. You could put them in alphabetical order or organize them into categories (sounds, feelings, etc.).

Word Art

You can also turn your new-found words into art. Instead of just writing your new words in your dictionary or for your word jar, you could create illustrations to go with your new words. Draw a picture of the meaning around the word.

Joanne Baker-Smith is an elementary school teacher, health & wellness coach, and author. She has taught in the NYC public school system for over 12 years. It was within this time, as an early childhood educator, where she began to notice areas and situations that made her young students feel concerned about their abilities. To help them, she utilized strategies to empower her students and give them confidence in their learning. It is these strategies that inspired Joanne's creation of the Little Learner Series to help children beyond her classroom feel as good about learning as her own students did. She lives in Forest Hills, New York with her husband and two children.

John Moorer; born in New York City, and raised on a steady diet of comic books, music, and philosophy. His favorite forms of art include traditional watercolors, acrylics, and both physical and digital sketching. With a love of the human figure and a passion for storytelling, you can usually find John writing or drawing something around his home in Long Island, New York.

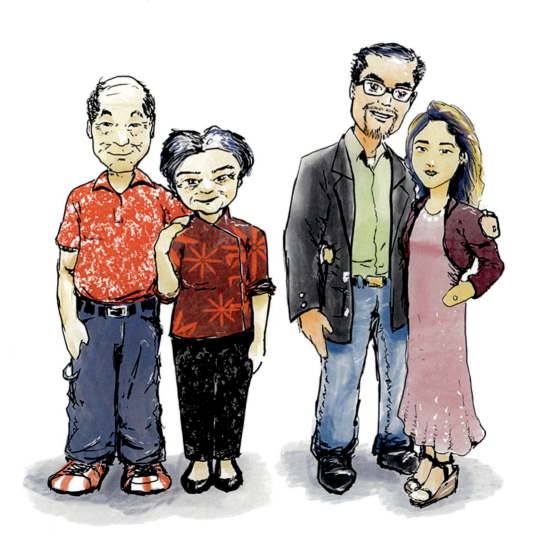

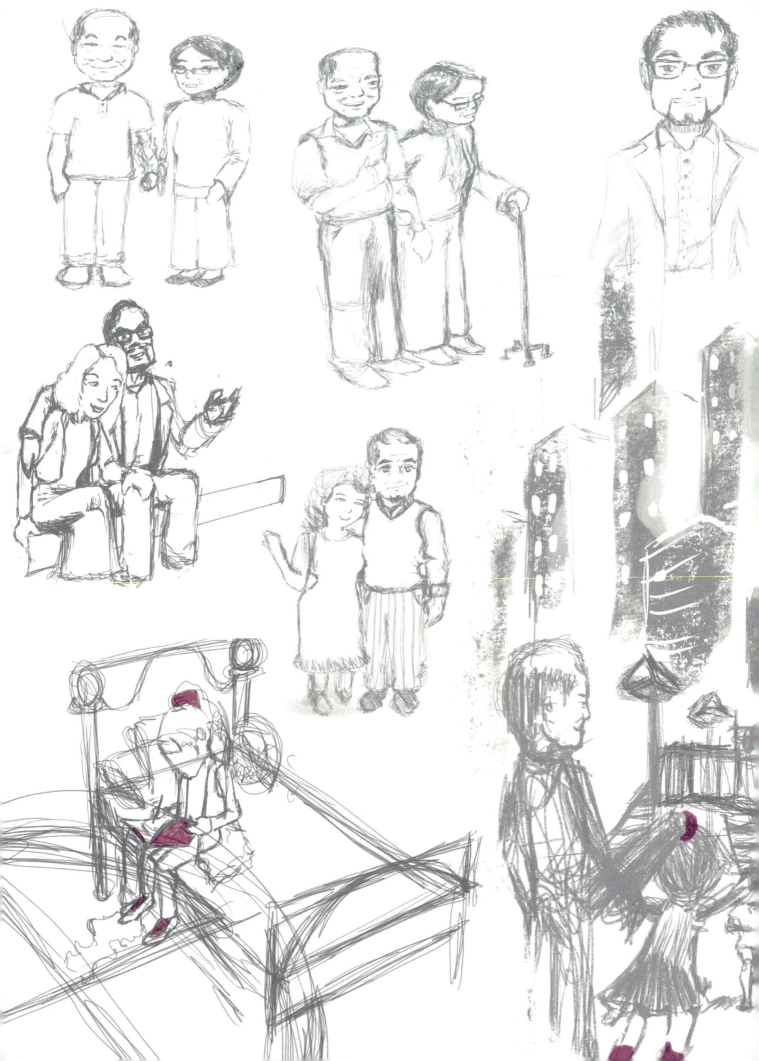

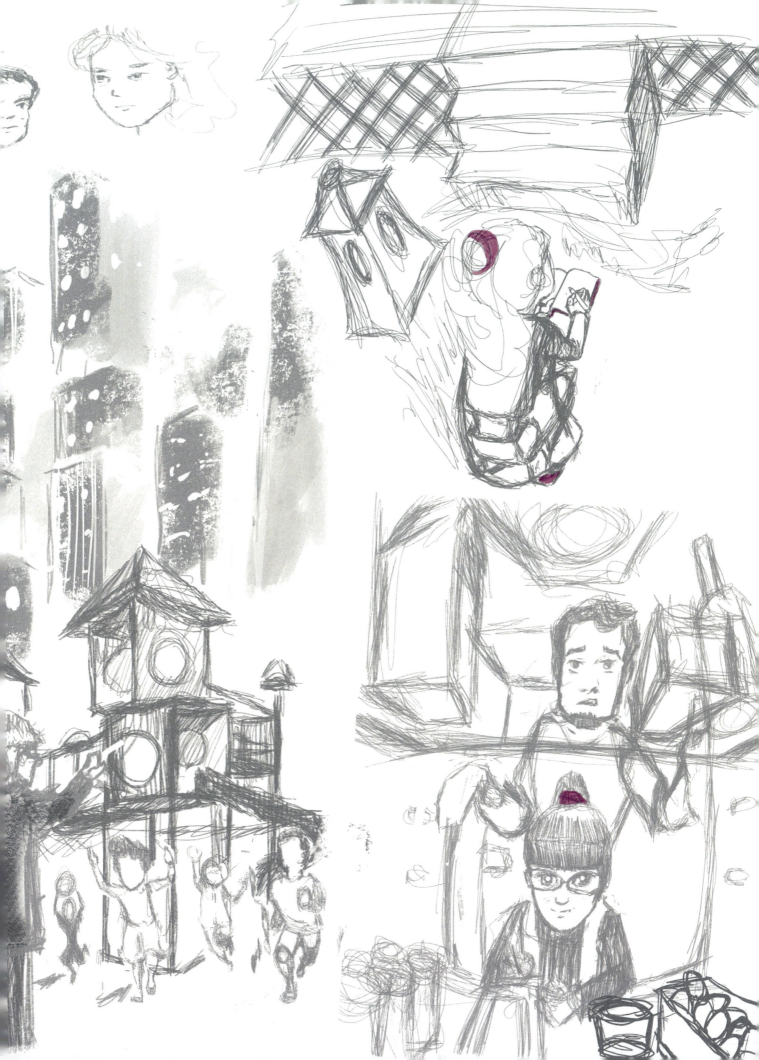

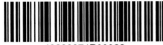

Made in the USA
Middletown, DE
20 June 2019